A STEP-BY-STEP GUIDE
TO BREASTFEEDING

A STEP-BY-STEP GUIDE TO BREASTFEEDING

CHRISTINA SIEGEL, MD

nurse-*well*

A STEP-BY-STEP GUIDE TO BREASTFEEDING

ISBN   978-1-5445-0081-2 *Paperback*

   978-1-5445-0044-7 *Ebook*

CONTENTS

ACKNOWLEDGMENTS

I want to thank some very talented people for their help and encouragement. Whitney Abbott for her beautiful illustrations. Ruth Hegarty for her time editing. Dr. Susan Shapiro for her vast knowledge and constant support. Robyn Van Tuyl whose talents abound. Layla Bayet for her hands-on support from day one. My family, my loving husband and my adorable son for always believing in me.

AUTHOR'S NOTE

Dear Nursing Mother,

By choosing to nurse, you are providing the best and healthiest form of nutrition for your baby. In studies, breastfed babies score higher on IQ tests, have fewer infections, and less chronic diseases. For making the choice to breastfeed, you should congratulate yourself.

With these wonderful benefits comes a challenge for you and your body to become proficient with nursing. At times, like I have, you may find discomfort or even pain from this very natural process, but these are usually short-term and after your third week of nursing, you should feel confident and comfortable with your abilities.

In the middle of the 20th century, worldwide breastfeeding decreased substantially, but times have changed and breastfeeding is now on the rise. Through education and progressive legislation, Scandinavia has led the comeback with 97 percent of all mothers attempting to nurse. Here in the U.S., we still have a way to go. I hope that by helping you make it through the first three weeks, you will have the knowledge and confidence to continue breastfeeding as long as you and your baby wish.

Wishing you the best of luck and the happiest of children!

Sincerely,

CHRISTINA SIEGEL, M.D.

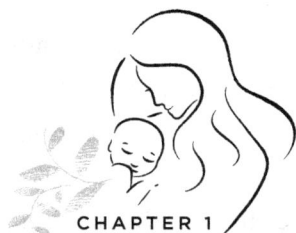

CHAPTER 1

INTRODUCTION

This is a survival guide to breastfeeding. It will serve as a guide for your first weeks of breastfeeding and as a nursing reference into the future. It is based both on my findings as a physician and my experiences as a nursing mother. The guide outline follows alongside your bodily changes and your baby's needs for the first three weeks after birth. There are a countless number of questions that arise during this time of discovery, and I have allotted a section of questions and answers (FAQs) pertaining to each week. These FAQs can server as a reference for questions throughout your entire nursing experience.

Each mother is unique, and your milk production may not follow the exact amounts referenced in this guide. Remember that your breasts haven't read the book! I have tried to keep all quantities in rough amounts (except where a universal statement is beneficial) to avoid excessive comparison to your particular situation and "the average." Use common sense and contact your physician or lactation consultant for any concerns.

In the text, I refer to you, the mother, directly and use 'her' or 'she' when speaking of your child regardless of the gender.

BENEFITS OF BREASTFEEDING

The medical experts all agree that no other infant food measures up to your breast milk.

They have proved that breastfeeding:

- Provides antibodies to a baby's developing immune system.
- Reduces incidence of diarrhea, upper-respiratory, ear infections, and many bacterial and viral illnesses.
- Protects against developing allergies, asthma, chronic digestive disorders, cardiovascular disease, diabetes, and eczema.
- Provides a stronger response to immunization.
- Provides hormones such as D.H.A.— important to brain and eye development.

- Decreases the risk of childhood cancer.

And for the mother, breastfeeding:

- Decreases risk of osteoporosis.
- Speeds postpartum healing of the uterus.
- Enhances mother-child attachment.
- Promotes weight loss.
- May reduce risk of ovarian and breast cancers.

HOW BREASTFEEDING WORKS

When you hit your third month of pregnancy, your hormones get to work on building up the milk ducts in your breasts. By the time you are six months' pregnant, your body is able to make breast milk, making sure that even if your child surprises you by coming early, you'll be ready for her.

You will find that your nipples will become exquisitely sensitive to touch. When your baby's mouth touches your nipple, nerve cells send a signal to your brain, causing the release of the hormone oxytocin. Oxytocin causes your uterine muscles to contract which is a benefit after labor. It also causes the tiny muscles within your breasts to contract, squeezing milk from milk-producing cells down the ducts towards the nipple. This is the *let-down reflex*.

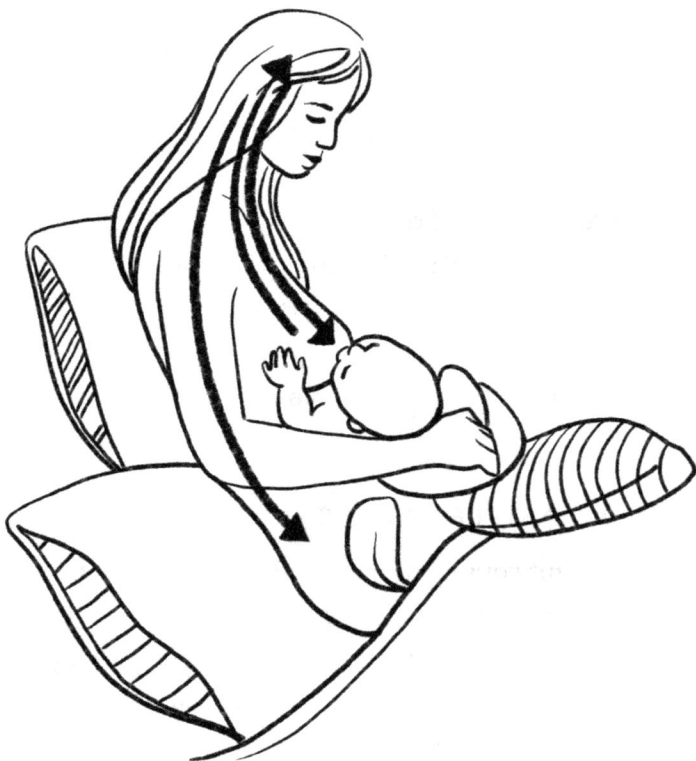

When your baby is correctly positioned and suckling at the nipple, we say the baby is **latched on**. As long as your baby is latched on, the amount of milk you produce is determined by how much your baby nurses. The more milk she drinks, the more your body will produce, and conversely, the less she drinks the less milk is produced. Your body works to match your production with your baby's needs.

Producing milk draws resources from your body. If your

diet contains insufficient nutrients for both you and your nursing child, your child will come first. This means that your breast milk will stay highly nutritious, but may leave your body nutritionally depleted. In this guide, we will look at all aspects of ensuring proper nutrition through preparation and education.

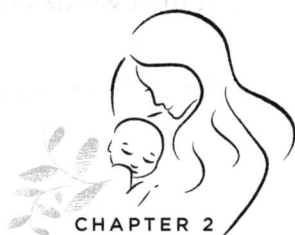

CHAPTER 2

BEFORE THE BIRTH

PREPARATION FOR NURSING

Like any new activity, the more you know about nursing, the better off you are to approach it successfully. We are going to look at preparation in two parts: physically constructing a comfortable environment for when you nurse and more importantly, preparing mentally for the months of nursing ahead.

As a trained physician, I was surprised by the amount of information I learned through working with midwives and experienced mothers. I received valuable guidance from my midwives—who talked at length about what a shock to the system nursing can be. I didn't take on board the true significance of their words until long after my baby was born. To aid new mothers, I now recommend planning for nursing alongside the development of your plans for birth.

THE NURSING PLAN

Nursing is going to be a totally new experience for you and your baby. Start before the birth by thinking about the experience as a whole. You can make a nursing plan at the same time you make a birth plan.

At the beginning, you are going to be nursing for up to eighteen hours a day, so you need to make this as pleasant an experience as possible. Set up a 'nursing station' in the living room and the bedroom or other suitable place of your choice. Get all the supplies you will need together so you don't have to move once you get settled: pillows, diapers, change of clothes, towel or cloth diaper for leaks or spit-up, breast pads, wipes, **water**, remote control, book to read, small snack, pen, paper and whatever else you might need.

To construct a nursing plan, consider the environment you would like to have while nursing. You may want to try out your desired location with nursing aids in place to make sure you can sit or rest with good posture for extended periods. Trial and error with cushions will help you establish the best environment, but remember, once nursing begins, you will not be able or wish to move.

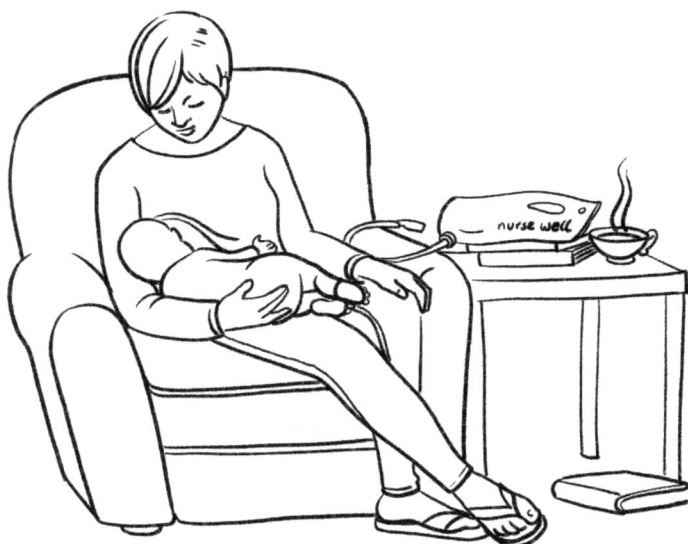

Above all, you need to have water by your side. The feeling of thirst initiated by your baby's suckling is intense and is Mother Nature's way of telling the body to replenish the water supply. It is recommended that the nursing mother drink twice that of the normal daily intake, thus, sixteen cups a day or a total of 128 ounces in twenty-four hours.

A nursing mother produces thirty-nine ounces of milk

per day (less as a newborn), containing 330 milligrams of calcium per quart. You are really feeding two people, and you use an average of 500 extra calories per day. Good nutrition is therefore just as important for you as it is for your baby.

You should also consider whether you want to have direct access to your baby immediately after giving birth. Your desires should be reflected in both your nursing and birth plan. I wholeheartedly recommend attempting to nurse from the moment your baby is born if it is possible in your particular situation.

Your baby is born with a suckling instinct, which she uses to learn how to nurse. This instinct is most intense immediately after birth, so it is best to introduce the breast within the first hour of life. The added benefit to you is that the suckling will also cause your uterus to contract and decrease the chance of excessive bleeding after delivery.

If possible, your baby should be allowed to "room in" which just means she sleeps next to you instead of in the hospital nursery. You should tell the nurses you wish to breastfeed on demand and would like to have your baby beside you as much as possible.

There is no evidence that mothers who are separated

from their babies are better rested. On the contrary, they are more rested and less stressed when they are with their babies. Mothers and babies learn how to sleep in the same rhythm. When the baby starts waking for a feeding, the mother is also starting to wake up naturally. Thus, it is often best if the baby is within easy reach, close to her mother.

MY NURSING PLAN

I will start nursing immediately after my baby is born. I will make sure I have **two pillows**—one for my back and one for underneath the baby available after birthing. I will bring the following items with me to the place of birth (hospital, home, or birthing center):

- My nurse-wellTM ready with two liters of mineral water.
- An organic, baby-safe nipple cream for application after each nursing session to prevent dry cracked nipples.
- My nursing snack (i.e., dried fruit or nuts).
- A book to read while nursing or my favorite CD.
- A handful of 'burp-cloths' or towels to clean up any mess.
- Clean, natural fiber breast pads and nursing bra.
- A comfortable nursing top.

When I return home, I will keep the same items available at my nursing station. This station will be in my favorite rocking chair where I can rest and relax with my baby. This location is for our use only, and I feel comfortable leaving my nursing aids here. I will arrange a back-support pillow to keep my back in proper alignment, and I will use a footstool to keep my feet up.

I will speak to my friends and relatives before the birth and make sure they review my plan with me so they will learn my needs during the first weeks of nursing and be able to fully support my baby and me.

This was my own personal nursing plan, and I encourage you to use it as a template for your own. A nursing plan is just as personal as a birthing plan. Devoting an equal amount of time to each plan will help you get off to a good start. This will save you time and energy after the birth when both are at a premium.

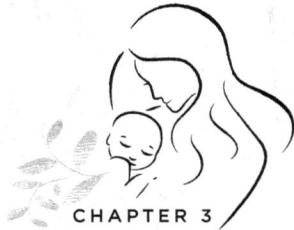

CHAPTER 3

WEEK ONE

You have readied your nursing plan, your beautiful bundle of joy has arrived, and now it is time for the first feeding. When you start making mature milk, we say your milk has *come in*. During the first few days, your milk has not yet *come in*; however, you are producing a special type of milk, called *colostrum*. Colostrum is a thick, yellow milk that is high in protein and boosts your baby's immune system. It may not look like the milk you are expecting—and you will only produce a small quantity. Do not worry. Your baby will only take in a few ounces per day of any milk throughout the first week.

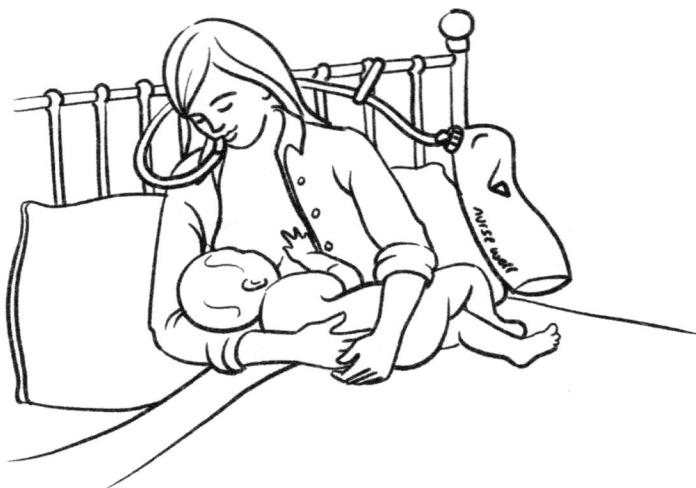

The first three days after birth are of particular importance for your baby to breastfeed. Besides the benefits of colostrum, your breasts are softer, (not yet *engorged*, or hardened with the pressure of milk inside) and it is easier for you and the baby to practice latching on. If you take advantage of this time, you can work with your baby on becoming skilled at breastfeeding for when your milk does come in and you start feeding for greater lengths of time.

Regardless of when you have the first opportunity to nurse, the first feeding is a time that deserves special attention.

THE FIRST FEEDING

The first time you nurse your baby, you may feel awkward, but like any skill, you will soon become proficient and confident at breastfeeding. A proper latch is crucial to success. A poor latch can cause sore nipples, and your baby may become inefficient and frustrated at feeding. Follow these steps to ensure that you and your baby get off to a good start.

Step 1. Position your baby on her side so she is directly facing you, with her belly touching yours—***belly-to-belly***.

Step 2. Using both hands, bring your baby to your breast. Try not to move your breast to the baby as this encourages bad posture.

Step 3. Place your thumb and fore-finger around your areola (the dark area around the nipple).

Step 4. Touch your baby's chin and upper lip to your nipple.

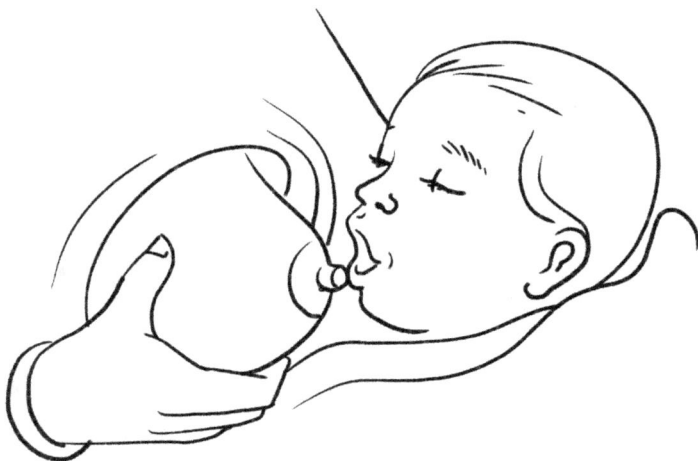

This will stimulate your baby's instinctual ability to search for food known as the ***rooting reflex***. She will open her mouth wide, as if yawning, and turn towards your breast.

Step 5. While her mouth is wide open, place as much as possibly of the areola into her mouth and tilt the top of her head towards your chest so she latches on.

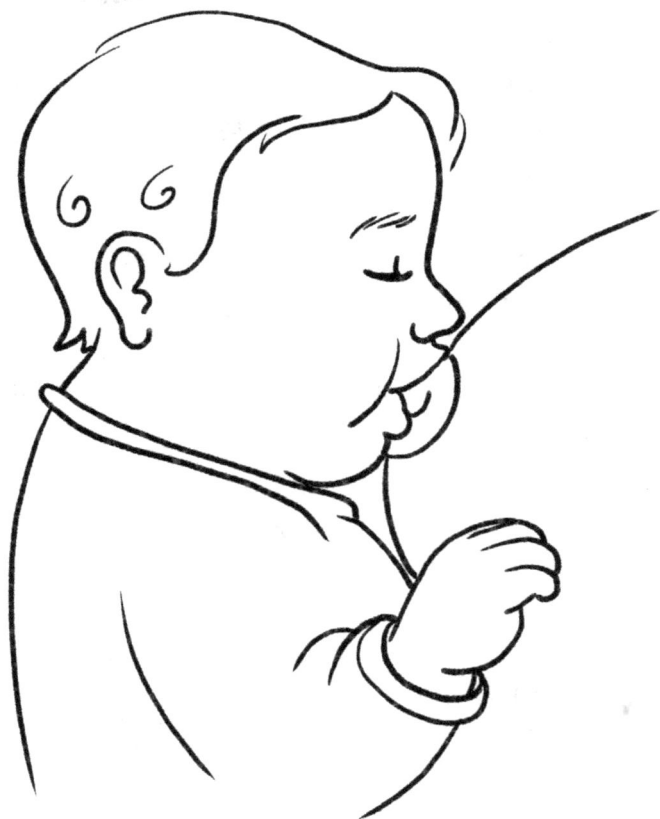

If the latch is good, she will start compressing her lips around the areola and sucking at first rapidly and then more rhythmically as the milk or colostrum lets down. Don't worry about her breathing. If she has trouble, she will pull away from the breast.

Step 6. If she comes off remember to start from the beginning again and remember to allow her to open her mouth as wide as she can before she takes the nipple.

By following these steps, you should have the necessary technique to have your baby latched-on in a position that reduces any irritation of the nipple. During the first few sessions, you will likely have many things on your mind, but it is important to check that your baby's lower lip does not get sucked into her mouth. It should stay in place around the areola.

Until you are confident that the baby is latched correctly, use your index finger to pull down on your baby's chin. This will ensure her lower lip remains out and in the correct position.

Before you leave the hospital, you should be shown that your baby is latched on properly, and that she is actually getting milk from the breast.

When you return home with your baby, she will help you learn her needs. Long before she starts crying, she will display signs that she is ready to feed. Her breathing will start to change, she will start to stretch or flex her body, and she will open her mouth wide. These are all signs of her rooting reflex. If the baby is sleeping with you, you will likely be especially in-tune with her breathing and movements.

During the first week, your baby will be asleep for many hours throughout the day. When your baby is awake and rooting, it is time to head to your nursing station and start breastfeeding.

WHEN YOUR MILK COMES IN

Two to five days after the birth, the colostrum will give way to a higher volume of transitional milk. At this time, we say that your milk has *come in.* Your breasts will become fuller, and it can be more difficult for the baby to get the whole of the areola in her mouth. This may make it difficult to keep your baby latched-on correctly. If you express a little milk first, the reduced tension can make it easier for your baby to latch on.

As your baby becomes more proficient, you may notice a *pins and needles* sensation after she latches on. This is the *let-down reflex*. You may also notice milk dripping or spurting from the other breast, and you should be prepared with extra towels and breast pads. You will also experience the urge to drink as soon as your milk lets down and you should be ready for this and drink from your Nurse-Welltm adlib.

The combination of sharply increased demand and increased supply can make you feel like you are nursing all the time. Daytime feedings may be less than two hours apart and last anywhere from ten minutes to an hour. Over time, feedings will continue to change in frequency and length depending on your baby's needs.

Alternative methods of getting your breast milk to your baby are available even if you are not always available to give it directly. A manual or electric breast pump allows storage of milk for use at a later date.

During the first week, there is usually no reason to restrict the frequency or length of your breastfeeding sessions. A sample schedule for your first week may look like this:

Day One

Let your baby decide – all day if she wants but your milk won't be in yet so try five minutes on one breast, then change to the other for another five minutes

Day Two

Again, your baby will be deciding but try putting her to the breast every two hours for ten minutes each side this time.

Day Three

Sit in your chosen nursing spot every three hours and aim for fifteen minutes on each breast.

Day Four

You should both be experts now and are ready to do: single-side feeding every three hours approximately and for a maximum of forty minutes.

Fifth Day-Seventh Day: Like the fourth day, but now start focusing on your posture and the position of your baby. Make sure her latch is strong and experiment with different positions.

Remember, this is a loose outline purely for guidance, and whatever routine works for you is the one you should stick with!

FAQ - WEEK ONE

Q. I have tried and tried to nurse, but my baby keeps biting my nipple when I am nursing. It hurts so much, I don't want to nurse. What can I do?

A. You will find that many difficulties during the first week of nursing arise from a poor latch. If your baby's mouth does not cover a good portion of your areola as well as your nipple, you will find the baby can easily fall out of a good latch. With the nipple fully in place in your baby's mouth, it is not easy for your baby to bite. Only when her mouth slips down around the nipple itself will she bite. Try to reset your baby's position and follow through the initial breastfeeding steps focusing on putting as much of the areola as possible into her mouth.

Q. How can I avoid sore nipples?

A. The number one cause of sore nipples is a poor latch. If you are being told your baby's latch is good despite having very sore nipples, be skeptical, and ask for help from a specialist. A lactation consultant, midwife or your local La Leche League group will be able to help you with specific difficulties.

Q. Do I have to sit in a chair to breastfeed?

A. No. Many mothers find it comfortable and even relaxing to breastfeed while lying down. This can be done if you lay on one side and position the baby, again belly-to-belly and follow the same procedures you would otherwise. It is even common to feed your baby side by side in the hospital. This is a great way for mothers to rest while the baby nurses.

Q. Once my baby starts crying, she will not take the breast. What can I do?

A. A baby who has been crying for some time before introducing the breast, may refuse to latch on even if she is ravenous. Babies often become frustrated and will not know how to calm themselves in their first week. Once she is crying, it is best to try calming her through other methods (i.e., rocking, speaking to her calmly, etc.). The moment she seems to be calming, reintroduce the breast and encourage her to latch on. This can be frustrating for you, but you will have a greater chance of success staying cool and calm.

Q. Does my baby need supplements of water or sugar water?

A. Unless directed by a medical professional, your baby will not need water or sugar water supplements. At birth, a baby's kidneys are not fully mature and water or sugar water alone are not suitable for your baby to digest. Breastmilk is the ideal fluid for your baby from birth.

Q. Does my baby need supplements of formula?

A. If you are breastfeeding several hours each day and you are lactating normally, supplementing with formula is unnecessary. If you have specific concerns about your milk production, you should seek consultation with a medical professional.

Q. Are my baby's bowel movements normal?

A. For the first few days after delivery, the baby passes *meconium*, a dark green, almost black substance. By the third day, the bowel movements start becoming lighter. Usually by the fifth day, the bowel movements have taken on the appearance of normal breast milk stool. Normal breast milk stool is pasty to watery, mustard colored, and usually has little odor. Bowel movements, however, may vary considerably from this description. They may be green or orange, may be lumpy or sticky, or may have air bubbles. The variation in color does not mean something is wrong. A baby who is breastfeeding only, and is starting to have bowel movements that are becoming lighter by day three of life, is doing well. A baby who is still passing meconium on the fourth or fifth day of life, should be seen by a physician that day.

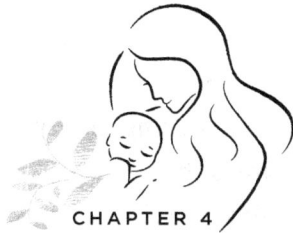

CHAPTER 4

WEEK TWO

IS MY BABY GETTING ENOUGH MILK?

During the second week, your baby's milk intake will likely become your focused. When your baby is born, she will be weighed and everyone will be talking about her birth weight. In the first week after birth, it is normal for your baby to lose on average eight ounces. This is no cause for alarm, and by the end of the second week, your baby should have regained this weight.

There are many ways you can observe your baby's milk intake. By the second week, your baby's bowel movements will have transitioned to breast milk stool (see FAQ - Week One). During the second week, other characteristics will provide more insight into how much milk your baby is receiving.

Your baby's nursing is characteristic. A baby who is obtaining good amounts of milk at the breast sucks in a very characteristic way. When a baby is getting milk (she is not getting milk just because she has the breast in her mouth and is making sucking movements), you will see a pause at the point of her chin after she opens to the maximum and before she closes her mouth, so that one suck is "open mouth wide, pause, close mouth." If you wish to demonstrate this to yourself, put your finger in your mouth and suck as if you were sucking on a straw. As you draw in, your chin drops and stays down as long as you are drawing in. When you stop drawing in, your chin comes back up. This pause to swallow that is visible at the baby's chin represents a mouthful of milk. The longer the pause, the larger the mouthful. A baby who does this type of sucking for twenty minutes straight is getting plenty of milk. One who nibbles for twenty hours will come off the breast hungry.

Another good indicator that your baby is getting sufficient milk is through monitoring her urination. With six soaking wet (not just wet) diapers in a twenty-four-hour period, during the second week of life, you can be sure that the baby is getting a lot of milk (if she is only breastfeeding). Unfortunately, the new super dry "disposable" diapers often feel dry even when full of urine, but when soaked with urine, they are heavy. The baby's urine should be almost colorless after the first few days, though occasional darker urine is not of concern.

GOOD HYDRATION

You should drink according to **your** thirst. Some mothers feel they are thirsty all the time, but others only while nursing. Your body knows if you need more fluids and makes you feel thirsty. You should however be aware of the amount you are drinking each day, as running low on fluids will only have adverse effects for you, the mother.

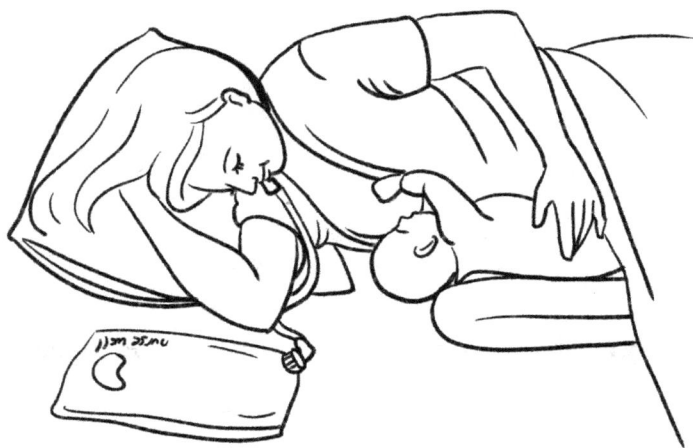

Dehydration, or lack of water, can leave you feeling terrible just when you need to be your strongest. Beware of symptoms like headache and fatigue, which are often caused and certainly made worse by lack of fluid intake.

It is recommended that every healthy adult drink eight glasses of water a day, but the nursing mother may need up to twice this amount. Your Nurse-WellTM holds eight of these eight-ounce glasses of water: enough for at least twelve hours. Be aware that caffeine and beer act as diuretics that will cause greater water loss. You need to account for this and compensate.

Healthy drinks that will replace your fluid losses include:

- Water
- Vegetable juice (natural)
- Soup (from fresh vegetables)
- Fruit juice (natural)
- Milk
- Herbal nursing tea

FAQ - WEEK TWO

Q. My baby seems to feed for hours and still appears hungry. What can I do?

A. A baby who drinks well will not be on the breast for hours at a time. Thus, if she is, it is usually because she is not latching on well and not getting the milk that is available. Get help to improve the baby's latch.

Q. Since I started nursing, I have frequent headaches and dry skin. Is there anything I can do about it?

A. Symptoms of fluid depletion that you should watch for include headache, fatigue, dry skin and mucous membranes. If you have these symptoms, your body can be in need of as much as two and a half liters of fluid immediately.

Should you get to the stage where you are dizzy when standing or changing position or your urine is a dark straw color and decreased in volume, your body can be in need of as much as six liters of fluid.

As both you and your baby are relying on the water YOU take in, it is very important to ensure an adequate supply both day and night. Remember, your baby is feeding just as much during the night as in the day, and because it is unlikely you will be eating much at night, it is even more critical you drink your water.

Q. My breast is hard, hot, and swollen. What can cause this and what can I do about it?

A. These are the typical symptoms of engorgement. To help ease these symptoms, wrap the breast in a hot, wet cloth. Then follow this exercise: Raise the hand on the side of the affected breast above your head and rotate your arm from the shoulder five times. Repeat every thirty minutes. **Consult your physician or midwife if the condition doesn't improve within twenty-four hours.**

Q. My breast is hard, hot, swollen and I have a fever, chills and night sweats. What can cause this and what can I do about it?

A. These symptoms may be caused by mastitis. Mastitis is a bacterial infection of the breast that can occur in breastfeeding mothers. As with almost all breastfeeding problems, a poor latch, and thus, poor draining of the breast sets up the situation where mastitis is more likely to occur. If the mother has symptoms consistent with mastitis for more than twenty-four hours, she should start antibiotics. Continue breastfeeding, unless it is just too painful to do so. If you cannot, at least express your milk as best you can in the meantime. Restart breastfeeding as soon as you are up to it, the sooner the better. Continuing breastfeeding helps mastitis to resolve more quickly. There is no danger for the baby. Remember the following tips:

- Contact your doctor/healthcare provider.
- Heat (warm towel or heating pad), applied to the affected area helps healing.

- Rest helps fight off infection.
- Fever helps fight off infection. Treat fever if it makes you feel bad, not just because it is there.
- Medication (acetaminophen, ibuprofen) for pain can be very good. You will feel better and the amount that gets to the baby is insignificant. Acetaminophen is probably less useful as it does not have an anti-inflammatory effect.

Abscess occasionally complicates mastitis. You will need to see a specialist for immediate treatment.

Q. I have a lump in my breast that is sore to touch. What can cause this and what can I do about it?

A. These are the typical symptoms of a blocked milk duct. During the time the block is present, the baby may be fussy when nursing on that side, as milk flow may be slower than usual, probably due to pressure causing collapse of other ducts. Blocked ducts can be made to resolve more quickly by:

Step 1. Continuing breastfeeding on the affected side.

Step 2. Draining the affected area better. One way of doing this is to position the baby so her chin "points" to the area of hardness. Thus, if the blocked duct is in the outside, lower area of your breast (about 4 o'clock), the football hold would be best. Another way of getting better draining of the breast is using breast compression while the baby is feeding—getting your hand around the blocked duct and using steady pressure.

Step 3. Applying heat to the affected area (with a heating pad or hot water bottle, but be careful not to injure your skin by using too much heat for too long a period of time).

Step 4. Try to rest. (Not always easy, but take the baby to bed with you.)

Step 5. Massage your breast using small circular motions around the lump and stroke towards the nipple. You won't actually see the milk come out but the lump should disappear within twelve hours.

Step 6. If untreated, this can lead to mastitis.

If you have a lump that is not going away or getting smaller over more than a couple of weeks, you should see a specialist.

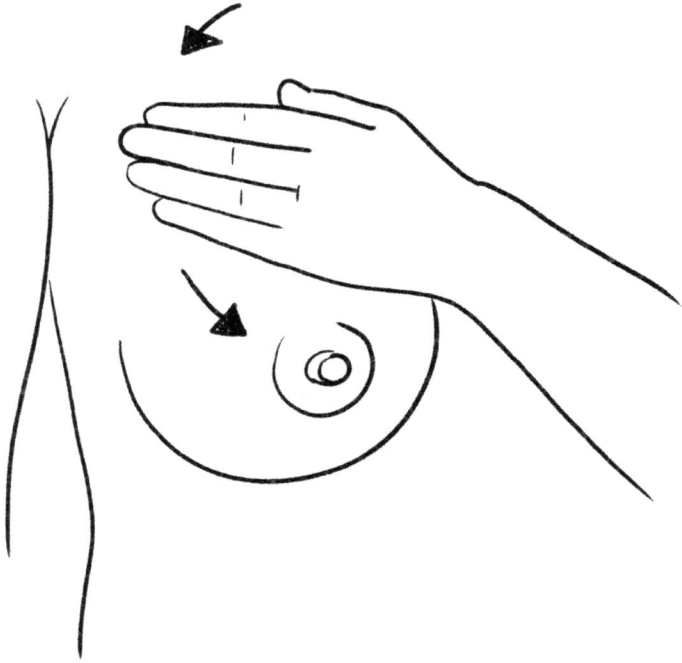

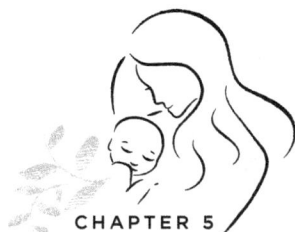

CHAPTER 5

WEEK THREE+

By the third week of breastfeeding, you should start to feel comfortable nursing your baby. You will know when your baby is hungry and it is wonderful to be able to satisfy her needs. At the beginning, you have many things to think about, and the most important factor is you and your baby finding techniques that work and feel good.

You have seen your milk change from colostrum when your baby was first born, to the mature milk you now have. You may also have noticed that the type of milk you produce changes from when your baby starts a feeding to when she finishes. The thin, almost clear milk that you first produce is called *foremilk*. Your baby will take in foremilk during most of a feeding. Towards the end of a good feeding, your breast will produce a thicker, creamy milk called *hindmilk*. This is very rich in calories and matches the needs of your baby's developing brain.

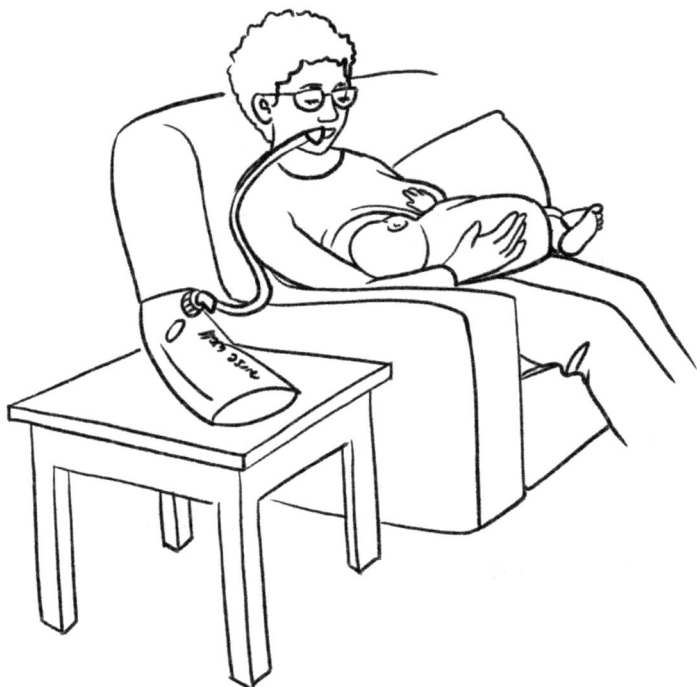

I recommend as you feel more confident nursing, letting your baby feed on one breast for an entire feeding—until she takes herself off the breast naturally. This allows her to benefit from the different types of milk your body is producing. You may find a rhythm that allows you to keep your baby on for an entire feeding, alternating breasts between each feeding.

GOOD NUTRITION

Eating a balanced diet provides your body with the nutrients it needs for breastfeeding and good health. According to the American Academy of Pediatrics, nursing mothers need to eat about 500 calories more each day. For most women, this means a total of 2,000 to 2,200 calories each day while breastfeeding.

Healthy eating is often not as easy as one would like. The American diet is rife with processed and refined foods—exactly the foods you should limit in a healthy diet. Instead, you should have whole grain foods at most meals and fats should come from those that are liquid, not solid at room temperature.

Vegetables should be eaten in abundance and organic are best for both you and your baby. A fruit serving two to three times a day is recommended and the same goes for nuts and legumes. Choose fish, poultry and eggs above red meat and butter. Moderation is the key to any healthy diet.

Your baby will tolerate most foods you normally eat. If you feel something you ate has upset the baby, then avoid that food. Write down your observations and consult with your physician or dietitian.

Maintaining your calcium intake while breastfeeding

and also throughout life will decrease your risk of osteoporosis. Make sure to get your calcium intake to at least 1,000mg a day.

Vegetarian diets should be taken very seriously. Pure vegetarians may not be getting all the necessary proteins and may have diets low in vitamin B12. Special diets should be continued only under the advice of a certified nutritionist or dietitian.

If there is something lacking in your diet, it will be your body that feels the effects first—not your baby's.

SOURCES OF CALCIUM	PROTEIN SOURCES	VITAMIN B12 SOURCES
Pre-natal vitamins	Tofu	Vitamin supplements
Broccoli	Beans combined	Fortified soy milk
Supplemental	with grains	Fortified yeast
Multivitamins	Eggs	Eggs
Dark green	Protein Shakes	
vegetables (except		
spinach)		
Calcium-fortified		
drinks		
Collards		
Rice		
Orange juice		
Cereals		
Tofu		
Salmon/Sardines		

MOTHERING THE MOTHER

Mothers today juggle more tasks, work longer hours and

sleep less than their own mothers did. Ways have to be found to cope with the relentless and sometimes overwhelming stresses of raising young children. The mother must be at her best for her family especially during the first years of her children's life when they are so dependent on her physically and emotionally. It is crucial to be prepared for this and to GET AS MUCH HELP AS POSSIBLE! Psychologists everywhere are now talking about DMS or Depleted Mother Syndrome as a new condition and it is a plague to our society. But treatment is simple: "mother the mother." Help the mother take care of herself so she can care for her family.

With this in mind, use breastfeeding as your ally. It is the best excuse in the world to take time out. Devote yourself to this one task as you should and let everyone around you worry about everything else. YOU are the only one who can breastfeed your infant and that is your job—a new job that will take all your concentration for at least the first six weeks. Ask anyone who starts a new job how long it takes to get comfortable and feel at ease with it. Everyone around you now has the job of supporting you in this very important role as mother.

Remember, nursing your baby is a job; don't plan to jump up as soon as you're done and run around doing errands.

You should be resting when your baby is resting and that means a nap for you both after every feed.

Good advice given to me by a very dear friend when I was pregnant was when people ask, give them a task. It can be as simple as bring the mail in from the mailbox or do a load of laundry. Your friends and family will be delighted to do this for you, and it is one less thing you have to think about.

Here is a list of chores for your wish list:

1. Do laundry.
2. Run dishwasher.
3. Sweep floor or vacuum.
4. Drop off milk, eggs, bread, cereal, etc.
5. Pick up baby wipes, diapers, baby shampoo, soap, extra burp clothes, breast pads, maternity pads, nice soap or bubble bath, etc.
6. Return library books.
7. Mow the lawn.
8. Replace a light bulb in the bathroom.

Your list is personal and can be as short or as long as you want. Remember, they don't all have to be chores; maybe at the top of your list should be a back rub! This is only the second time in your life when you get to be mothered; the first was when you were born!

Why not set up a food chain where all your friends and relatives get to bring you a meal during the first weeks after you've given birth? This can be organized at your baby shower or at least a month before your due date.

It works like this:

- Everyone gets a copy of a list with names and phone numbers in order.
- When the first person drops off food to you, they call the next person to tell them it's their turn and so on down the chain.
- Ask people to stay just long enough for a quick chat and to see your gorgeous baby before they leave you to enjoy your home-cooked treat.

You know you'll love to repay the favor when their time comes.

ADVICE FOR FAMILY AND FRIENDS

"It takes a village to raise a child."

–UNICEF

This is a very demanding time for your wife/daughter/ girlfriend and she needs your support more than ever before. Mothers can't succeed without support. Give her everything you think she will need, and more, to do this demanding job. This job is not nine to five or even near; it is twenty-four hours, seven days a week and both physically and emotionally very demanding. If she is struggling, let her know this is normal and you are available to help.

Do things without asking. Remember to add to the list of chores she would like done with treats she may appreciate receiving. Maybe a book by her favorite author is in order. If you can't be by her side, a phone call to say she is doing a good job and keep up the good work can make her day (makes a good answering machine message too).

If she is struggling at the beginning, discourage visitors and promote quiet time for just mother and baby to get to know each other. Help her keep track of progress by filling in her logbook for her and refilling her water every chance you get.

Remember not to be critical of how she is doing things. Now is a very sensitive time. Her hormones can also be causing her to be very weepy and bursts of tears for no particular reason are very normal at this time. You should even expect them and just remember to remain supportive; these too will pass.

My wonderful husband was very shocked when his

normally very levelheaded wife was sobbing and couldn't explain why. As a treat, he invited my two best friends from overseas to come and cheer me up. Remember, every woman is different and will respond differently to this life-changing event, so just be prepared. And if you are not sure what to do, you too can ask for help.

Have the name and number of a lactation consultant or midwife you trust in town at your fingertips for when you need it. If you are going to have guests or relatives staying at your house, you may want to make a sign for the nursing mother. Something to post on the door of her bedroom or whichever room she would like to use for her quiet nursing sanctuary. As an example:

"Behind this door: a new mother and her baby are getting to know each other for the first time. They are in the process of learning the new and challenging skill of nursing. In order to do this, they need all the peace, rest and relaxation you can afford them.

They would love you to visit but appreciate your consideration and ask you not to interrupt during feeding time. Remember to offer to refill mom's Nurse-Welltm with water or get her a snack."

You can, of course, customize this to fit **your** nursing

mother's own needs. Remember, the support and encouragement of family and friends can be very important for a successful mother-baby nursing relationship.

FAQ - WEEK THREE+

Q. Can I give my baby both breast and bottle?

A. Yes. Remember every baby has different learning curves for breastfeeding. It is commonly advised to introduce a bottle at three weeks as breastfeeding is usually well established by this time. If you want the baby to feed from both the breast and a bottle you will have to work hard to balance using both each day. Every baby is an individual and this transition to using two techniques for feeding may be more difficult for some babies.

Babies will take whatever gives them a rapid flow of fluid and may refuse others that do not. Thus, in the first few days, when the mother is normally producing only a little milk (as nature intended), and the baby gets a bottle from which he gets rapid flow, he will tend to prefer the rapid flow method. There seems to be some controversy about whether "nipple confusion" exists. Nipple confusion includes a range of problems; including the baby not taking the breast as well as he could and thus not getting milk well and/or the mother getting sore nipples from a poor latch. It can cause a lot of problems for both mother and baby. Get help if you need it.

Q. My baby's stool has changed. Is this related to my milk production?

A. Some breastfed babies, after the first three to four weeks of life, may suddenly change their stool pattern from many each day, to one every three days or even less. Some babies have gone as long as fifteen days or more without a bowel movement. As long as the baby is otherwise well, and the stool is the usual pasty or soft, yellow movement, this is not constipation and is of no concern.

Q. When is it time to consult my physician?

A. If your breasts are sore, you feel a burning sensation in them, and your baby has a diaper rash with spotty red skin. You may have a yeast infection and you should call your physician.

If you have a fever and your breasts are hot, tender and have uneven bright red lines across them, you may have mastitis. You should contact your physician.

Whatever problems you encounter don't hesitate to seek help. Your doctor will be able to address your concerns and can also refer you to a lactation consultant.

FINAL WORDS

By reading this guide and following the steps outlined, you should be off to a great start. If your interest has been piqued by a particular subject, I encourage you to continue your reading. There are larger, more comprehensive texts that go into great depth in each area. I have listed some of these in the Reference section at the end of this guide.

There are few roles in life that are as fulfilling as that of a nursing mother. With the knowledge and techniques you now have, you can continue nursing as long as you and your child desire. Your work and commitment has given you the opportunity to embrace this genuinely rewarding experience. I'm sure you will treasure yours as much as I do mine.

REFERENCES

1. The Economic Impact Of Breastfeeding. Ball TM - *Pediatr Clin North Am* - 01-FEB-2001; 48(1): 253-62

2. Breast-Feeding And The Onset Of Atopic Dermatitis In Childhood: A Systematic Review And Meta-Analysis Of Prospective Studies. Gdalevich M - *J Am Acad Dermatol* - 01-OCT-2001; 45(4): 520-7

3. Does the duration and frequency of early breast-feeding affect nipple pain? De Carvalho M, Robertson S, Klaus MH: Birth 11:81, 1984

4. Maternal weight-loss patterns during prolonged lactation. Dewey KG, Heinig MI, Nommsen LA: Am J Clin Nutr 58:162, 1993

5. Lactation and breast cancer risk. Furberg H, Newman B, Moorman P, et al: Int J Epidemiol 28:396–402, 1999

6. Studies of perceived milk insufficiency. Hillver-vick-Lindquist C, Hofvander Y, Sjolin S: Acta Paediatr Scand 80:297, 1991

7. Physiology of lactation. Lawrence RA, Lawrence RM: In Breastfeeding: A Guide for the Medical Profession, ed 5. St. Louis, CV Mosby Company, 1999, pp 59–94 1.

8. Breastfeeding- starting out right. Jack Newman, MD, FRCP. www.bflrc.com/newman

9. The frequency of suckling. A neglected but essential ingredient of breastfeeding. Klaus MH – Obstet Gynecol Clin North Am- 01 Sept – 1987 14(3); 623-33.

10. Medical complications of the mother. Lawrence RA, Lawrence RM: In Breastfeeding: A Guide for the Medical Profession, ed 5. St. Louis, CV Mosby Company, 1999, p 526

11. Diet and dietary supplements for the mother and infant. Lawrence RA, Lawrence RM: In Breastfeeding: A Guide for the Medical Profession, ed 5. St. Louis, CV Mosby Company, 1999, pp 297–334

12. Breast-feeding reduces maternal lower-body fat. Kramer FM - *J Am Diet Assoc* - 01-APR-1993; 93(4): 429-33

PARENTS ON BREASTFEEDING

"We all know the story of the exhausted mother or father staggering about in the middle of the night trying to prepare a bottle for a frantic child. By the time it's ready, the baby is so worked up she can't go back to sleep. None of that with breastfeeding, oh no. Night feeds are performed lying down in bed, latch him on and drift off - much more civilized. I think my husband found this very appealing as he was getting up for work at 6:00 a.m. feeling fresh as a daisy, while his 'new father' colleagues were staggering about with bean-bags under their eyes."

—ANN, MOTHER OF JAKE (AGE 2)

"Breastfeeding is very slimming! I regained my pre-pregnancy weight after three months. I eat what I like, chocolate, cakes, chips, pastries, and great big dinners! I have the metabolism of an athlete and 4000 calories a day has no effect on my thighs!"

—JULIE, MOTHER OF KIM (AGE 1)

"Breastfeeding will bond you with your baby in a way words can't explain. You don't know how many times I looked down at my daughter as she nursed and tears of joy fell on her face. What comfort she must have felt there so warm and secure in my arms at my breast."

—SUSAN, MOTHER OF EMMA (AGE 2)

ABOUT THE AUTHOR

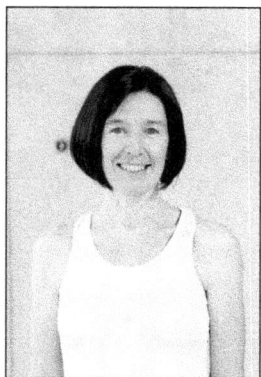

CHRISTINA SIEGEL, MD, CPT, is the founder and sole practitioner of Tea with the MD, a wellness planning practice. Dr. Siegel holds a medical degree from the Royal College of Surgeons and her training includes European and US medical care. Dr. Siegel is certified by the Athletics and Fitness Association of America and the National Academy of Sports Medicine and earned her spinning certification with spinning founder Jonathan Goldberg. Christina has lived in Santa Barbara, Las Vegas, San Francisco, Dublin, and Tokyo with her husband and a growing number of Irish-American children (currently eight).

www.ingramcontent.com/pod-product-compliance
Lightning Source LLC
Chambersburg PA
CBHW060521280326
41933CB00014B/3053